EMERGING FROM THE CURVE:

THE STUDENTS OF WEST VILLAGE ACADEMY
SHARE THEIR STORIES

Stories Compiled by
Angie BEE & Bartee Productions

A Written Adaptation of the
Confinement Chronicles Audiobook Series
with the Students of West Village Academy

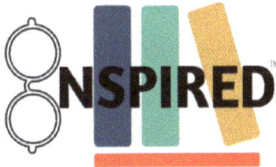

NSPIRED™

Reading for the Whole Person

INSPIRED published by
Ladero Press LLC
229 Kettering Road
Deltona, Florida 32725

First Ladero Press Printing, April 2021

Emerging from the Curve:
The Students of West Village Academy Share Their Stories

ISBN: 978-1-946981-75-2 Paperback / 978-1-946981-76-9 EPUB /
978-1-946981-77-6 Mobi

Printed in the United States of America
Set in Times New Roman
Cover Designed by SheerGenius

Scriptures taken from the Holy Bible, New International Version®, NIV®. Copyright © 1973, 1978, 1984, 2011 by Biblica, Inc.TM Used by permission of Zondervan. All rights reserved worldwide. www.zondervan.com The "NIV" and "New International Version" are trademarks registered in the United States Patent and Trademark Office by Biblica, Inc.TM

The *Inspired* logo is a trademark of Ladero Press.
The *Where Writers Can Soar* logo is a trademark of Ladero Press.

Library of Congress information available upon request.
www.laderopress.com

TABLE OF CONTENTS

AN INTRODUCTION FROM ME,
"DA QUEEN BEE"...
EVANGELIST ANGIE BEE

When the Lord first instructed me to produce an inspirational audiobook, I never dreamed that authors from far-and-wide would contribute to this project! As they continued to send us their stories, I slowly began to realize that all of these stories would not fit in a sixty-minute audio! Why the sixty-minute specification? Well, although we are now in the age of mp3 players, there are still people that want to listen to a compact disc, and CDs can hold up to sixty minutes of audio. I was thinking small; God showed me HIS bigger picture.

Soon, we had enough stories to fill Volume I, and even Volume II; and this was only May 20th! The posted deadline for submissions was June 1, 2020, and I was still waiting on contributions from three more people! LOOK AT GOD! Now, I understand that *Confinement Chronicles* will never end; just like the Word of God never grows old. The 2020 series included "Confinement Chronicles" of our minds and our relationships. There was a "Confinement Chronicles" of our finances and our "lack of faith." We wrote about the protests during the pandemic, the children affected by the pandemic, and so much more.

Now, with the 2021 series, we are focused on topics that are encouraging and uplifting, as we strive to "emerge" from this curve and find our "new normal", bringing us to this first volume. In one-way-or-another, these inspirational audiobooks will continue to encourage us to hear the Word of God, encourage us to write, and encourage us to share as they bring a historical record of how we survived the Pandemic of 2020.

Let me now tell you the story of some elite students that attend West Village Academy, a school in Michigan.

I was contacted on Facebook by a woman who saw a video that I did for a fellow author. The author's name is Vincent Taylor, and in the video, I read a portion of his children's book for The International GREAT Black Read Aloud Day, created by Ladero Press. You see, Ladero Press is a publishing company that created a day/week/month when people could log on to watch videos of people reading excerpts from books written by black authors. Well, I read a chapter from Mr. Taylor's book *Cornbread Faces the School Bully* and posted the video on Facebook. Ms. Carletta Counts saw the video, contacted me, and now her West Village Academy students are authors!

You see, The Lord had already developed and birthed a virtual writing workshop through me in preparation for these students. I had tested it out on family and a few adult authors, months earlier. The West Village Academy students were already working on their contribution to the *Confinement Chronicles* audiobook project, yet, the Lord instructed me to contact their after-school site coordinator about the virtual writing workshop. Michelle Khatib spoke with the school leaders, and they agreed to allow me to present this virtual workshop to these students! Just seeing their faces on camera warmed my soul as we discussed writing topics, composing a bio, and creating paragraphs --

all while listening to music! At the end of the ninety-minute session, I shed tears of completion and joy! Then, on March 1, 2021, when I received the email that contained their story submissions - - I gave God all the praise!

The team at Angie BEE Productions would like to give a special dose of gratitude to the following administration team members at West Village Academy:

1. Carletta Counts – CAO/Superintendent
2. Brad Miller – Building Principal
3. Ernestine Howard – Elementary Principal
4. Michelle Khatib – Site Coordinator, 21st CCLC After School Program
5. Carlen Ford – 21st CCLC After School Program Teacher
6. Michelle Hall – 21st CCLC After School Program Teacher
7. Lisabeth Mikolajczyk – 21st CCLC After School Program Teacher
8. Lottie Larkins – 21st CCLC After School Program Teacher

Without the support of these school leaders, inspiration from Ladero Press to read via video, and the enthusiasm of these students, you most certainly would not be enjoying this project.

Now, it's time for our first contribution …

EMERGING FROM THE CURVE:

THE STUDENTS OF WEST VILLAGE ACADEMY
SHARE THEIR STORIES

ERINAYO OLAYADE

I want to talk to you about the pandemic and the Coronavirus. We were all at home stuck doing our school work on the computers. It has really changed the way my day goes. I go to sleep earlier and wake up later. I can eat my lunch at home. I do my afterschool programs on the computer, and I learn a lot of stuff. What I like about what's happening is that I can spend more time with my family. I can sleep in later. I miss school, but it's good to stay safe and stop the coronavirus from spreading. I hope when I get to school, I can make more friends.

Bio

Hi, my name is Erinayo. I am nine years old. I am from West Village Academy in Dearborn, Michigan.

These next two contributions were narrated in the original audiobook by a member of "Da Bee Hive Intern Crew" at #DBHIC.
He is known as Jalen Bee, and he is a 9th grade student at Cass Technical High School in Detroit Michigan.

CHRISTIAN GLASS

This first story was written by Christian Glass. Christian was born June 22, 2008, in Hansel Hospital. He is 12 years old and in grade 7A. When asked what his recent goal is, he says: "I want to graduate college." Christian's future aspirations? "In the future," he says, "I want to be an astronaut, artist, and architect."

Christian's Story

During the virus, schools, stores, etc., were closed, and I felt really bad for the people who had the virus because the virus has now killed over 500,000 people, and the virus can be a really dangerous disease. My personal experience during the shutdown was good because I'm finally getting used to the Google meetings.

March, April, and May of 2020, I was doing my school work, and after I was done with my work, I watched TV, got on the tablet, phone, laptop, or PlayStation. June 2020, I was getting out of school, and the summer break was about to begin. July 2020, I was outside, riding my bike, playing video games, going to the store with my mom, and going everywhere else with mom.

I feel pretty confident about what I just wrote. I do feel bad about what is going on in the world now and for all the families that have lost their loved ones during these difficult times--and just praying for better days because we're all in this together.

The End

DELLONDOE WILLIAMS

This next story comes from Dellondoe Williams, a 9-year-old resident of Westland, Michigan.

My Life During the Pandemic

When the pandemic started and the Governor shut down the state, I was at my dad's. I live with my mom, but since she is a frontline worker for Henry Ford, she thought I was safer with my dad. I stayed with my dad for a month. My mom and granny were very sad and missed me, and they cried a lot. At my dad's, it was me, my older sister, my dad, and grandma. We had a lot of fun together. We played board games like Checkers, and card games like Match.

After a month, I spent a weekend with my mom. We played games like Dino Operation and Uno, and we had an Easter egg hunt -- that was the best part. My mom had the best hiding spots; Granny and I couldn't find all her eggs. We didn't like that. I was very sad to leave; I wanted to stay. But my mom thought it was safe for me to go.

Both my parents decided that weekends would be better so my mom and granny wouldn't be so sad. Eventually, my schedule changed again to one week with my dad and the other with my mom. I thought it was fair since I enjoyed seeing my mom and granny more often.

A few months later, my mom fell down some stairs and hurt her shoulder, so I was home for three weeks before I went back to my dad's. My mom bought the coolest games: tabletop foosball, Pin Ball, and Plumbers Pants game. But my favorite game was a word search game. My mom and I had a challenge with the Pin Ball game, and I won. My prize was Burger King, but if I lost, I would have had to vacuum. It's pretty funny since vacuuming is one of my chores anyway, so maybe, it wasn't a challenge. We just had a lot of fun.

The End

This next contribution was narrated in the original audiobook by a member of "Da Bee Hive Intern Crew" at #DBHIC.

She is known as Sandra Bee, and she is a 3rd grade student at PACE Academy in Southfield, Michigan.

KAEDYN FORD

My name is Kaedyn Ford. I am 11 years old, and I like dancing, history, writing, and crafts. I have a little sister, and she is two years old! My birthday is 3/7/09. I am going to be twelve soon!

Hello! My name is Kaedyn, and I will share my experience with you all.

The pandemic started when I had just turned 11 years old. At first, I was very happy that I didn't have to go to school. But when they told my family that we were gonna have to stay at home for a while, I didn't feel a certain way about it. Eventually, I started to see how it affected my family. My mom lost her car, and my dad had to get two more jobs. School got harder. Then, my close cousin caught Covid. She survived it, but it still scared me.

When I started school, that's when everything went south for me. The work kept coming. No matter how much I did, I felt like crying. I felt like I was a disappointment. I felt like no one would miss me if I were gone. I was literally crying myself to sleep. When I told my friends, some left me, and some helped me through it. My family became more angry and aggravated. And I was becoming more and more mean, as well. When I realized that, I literally became a bully. I later realized what I had become, and I said sorry to the people I had wronged.

All my family was suffering, and it pained me to see it. I felt like I did nothing to help. I felt like I was a burden. So, I would try to help out and watch the little kids in my family. I feel like I'm in a jail cell.

I feel trapped, and I can't escape because I'm scared of what the future holds for me.

The pandemic made everyone around me sad also because all the rappers and actors kept dying. The coronavirus has transformed life as we know it. Schools are closed; we're confined to our homes; and, the future feels very uncertain. We are living through history. Future historians may look back on the journals, essays, and art that ordinary people are creating now to tell the story of life during the pandemic.

But writing can also be deeply therapeutic. It can be a way to express our fears, hopes, and joys. It can help us make sense of the world and our place in it.

The End

JESUS TILLMAN

First of all, I just want to say that Covid 19 is still around, and please stay safe. Anyway, I want to tell you that Covid 19 messed up my life like a scar because I had it. It felt like my body was aching, and I kinda lost my taste a little bit. But I mostly didn't lose my taste or smell. It affected my travel life because, for a few weeks, everything was closed. So, I couldn't visit places like different states, but after months in quarantine, we got to go out to places, and I'm lucky I live in Detroit because we got to go to the Underground Railroad, the Abraham Lincoln chair, and view the slave chains.

When I was in school, I always wished that we were homeschooled, but now I kinda wish I didn't say that because it happened. Be careful about what you wish for, but I know you're wondering how I got Covid 19. Well, it's kind of a long story, so, here's the short version. I got it from a teacher. Then, I got my dad sick. So, that's how Covid 19 ruined my life. Wait, I didn't talk about 2020. Well, I lost a lot of relatives, my favorite actor, and basketball player.

So, that's that, and thank you for reading my book. Bye.

OUR NARRATORS

Our youth narrators for the audiobook are voice actors, trained by Angie BEE Productions to be a part of "Da Bee Hive Intern Crew - #DBHIC

They are each Michigan residents and also are contributing authors in the *Confinement Chronicles* audiobook series!

Jalen Alexander

Jalen Alexander is a 15-year-old Arts Studies student born and raised in Detroit, Michigan. Attending a college-prep high school, Jalen possesses many talents including the visual arts. He has mastered several musical instruments and has traveled extensively competing and excelling in the challenging sport of Chess.

Jalen is a son/brother/grandchild/nephew and a doting uncle that displays respect, a great sense of humor, and a sincerely nurturing spirit. He now holds the most auspicious title of Author in his inaugural contribution in the *Confinement Chronicles* series, expressing his thoughts and feelings about living through this pandemic. Jalen enjoys playing card games and video games, and thrilling his family with his magic tricks.

Contact Jalen at JSpice414@gmail.com

Sandra "Bee"

Sandra "Bee" is an 8-year-old third grader, born in Michigan. She has been an entrepreneur since seven. Sandra is a baptized member of Beth Eden Missionary Baptist Church in Detroit, and she is a trained voice actress/narrator with Angie BEE Productions.

Sandra has been featured in several national commercials and audiobooks, and she has even read books to her peers during outreach workshops! Follow Sandra online via Facebook at:

www.facebook.com/SandraBowBoss

ABOUT THE MUSIC IN THE AUDIOBOOK VERSION

T he background music that is heard in the audiobook version of *Emerging from the Curve: The Students of West Village Academy Share Their Stories* is produced by the incomparable Larry D. Boyd, also known as DJ Shyheim. I live in North Carolina, and this is where I am reputable for my professional Disc Jockey services. Check out my homepage for more detailed information about what I do. Keep reading the text provided on this page to get familiar with my story and how I became a DJ.

PROFESSIONAL AND RELIABLE WEDDING & BIRTHDAY PARTY DISC JOCKEY SERVICES IN NORTH CAROLINA

When I was in high school, I used to stay up late at night recording all the trending songs on the radio. I kept doing that until it became my profession. I have performed in Japan, Florida, and California, working with major artists such as Christian (on Roc-A-Fella

Records), and as a DJ for Goodie Mob, Bad Azz, and others.

I personally believe that bringing a different sound to the table is the most important part of the job. Artists should be taken aside and compared to others. This is what I offer here at Halftime Productions – a unique sound and professional Disc Jockey service suitable for every event.

WHY CHOOSE ME?

Nearly 20 years of Experience ~ Pure Dedication
Qualification ~ Professional Equipment ~ Reasonable Rates

CALL (919) 770-8993 WHENEVER YOU NEED OUR
PROFESSIONAL DISC JOCKEY SERVICE IN NORTH CAROLINA!

If you are planning a special event in or around the NC area and looking for an experienced DJ to contact, know that you are making the right choice with me. Call Halftime Productions now at (919) 770-8993 to check for availability!

Website: http://halftimeproductionsnc.com/
Email: shyheim_28@yahoo.com

Instagram
shyheim_28

Facebook
djshyheim

Twitter
djshyheim

The Vision Behind
Confinement Chronicles

Evangelist Angie BEE
"Da Queen Bee"

Confinement Chronicles, an inspirational Christian audiobook series, was inspired by the global pandemic of 2020. It includes contributions from several authors, and is published in audio file increments of sixty minutes each. Our supportive biblical scripture for this project comes from Psalm 9:9 which reads:

The Lord is a refuge for the oppressed, a stronghold in times of trouble. NIV

This project is arranged and led by Evangelist Angie BEE. The audiobook is published by Angie BEE Productions and narrated by "Da Queen Bee" Evangelist Angie BEE. Guest narrators from "Da Bee Hive Intern Crew - #DBHIC" are included.

Search for www.Facebook.com/ConfinementChroniclesByAngieBEEProductions

As more volumes are produced and more people become authors, you will receive updates and inspiration from the Facebook page at www.Facebook.com/ConfinementChroniclesByAngieBEEProductions. The audiobook listening tour launches in 2021, so, get ready to come out and meet the authors, shop with the vendors, learn from the presenters, and enjoy yourselves.

Some final thoughts from me … "Da Queen Bee"

During the pandemic, as COVID-19 and the mutant variants continue to plague our world in 2021, I encourage each of you to remain patient, look for innovative ways to remain encouraged, and above all - - STAY FOCUSED ON GOD'S PLAN FOR YOUR LIFE!

Special thanks to our promotional sponsors, Donna M. Gray-Banks and the F.R.E.S.H. Book Festival at https://www.freshbookfestivals.net and Theresa Jordan, founder of Triumphant Magazine on Facebook. Follow Angie BEE Productions on Facebook. Search for *Confinement Chronicles* by Angie BEE Productions on Facebook, visit us online at www.DaQueenBee.com or send an email to AngieBEEproductions@gmail.com

Check on your leaders, your family and your friends, keep writing, and BEE Blessed!

www.ingramcontent.com/pod-product-compliance
Lightning Source LLC
Chambersburg PA
CBHW052125030426
42335CB00025B/3114